Fast Mimicking Diet

A Beginner's 2-Week Step-by-Step Guide and Overview on FMD, With Sample Recipes

copyright © 2022 Bruce Ackerberg

All rights reserved No part of this book may be reproduced, or stored in a retrieval system, or transmitted in any form or by any means, electronic, mechanical, photocopying, recording, or otherwise, without express written permission of the publisher.

Disclaimer

By reading this disclaimer, you are accepting the terms of the disclaimer in full. If you disagree with this disclaimer, please do not read the guide.

All of the content within this guide is provided for informational and educational purposes only, and should not be accepted as independent medical or other professional advice. The author is not a doctor, physician, nurse, mental health provider, or registered nutritionist/dietician. Therefore, using and reading this guide does not establish any form of a physician-patient relationship.

Always consult with a physician or another qualified health provider with any issues or questions you might have regarding any sort of medical condition. Do not ever disregard any qualified professional medical advice or delay seeking that advice because of anything you have read in this guide. The information in this guide is not intended to be any sort of medical advice and should not be used in lieu of any medical advice by a licensed and qualified medical professional.

The information in this guide has been compiled from a variety of known sources. However, the author cannot attest to or guarantee the accuracy of each source and thus should not be held liable for any errors or omissions.

You acknowledge that the publisher of this guide will not be held liable for any loss or damage of any kind incurred as a result of this guide or the reliance on any information provided within this guide. You acknowledge and agree that you assume all risk and responsibility for any action you undertake in response to the information in this guide.

Using this guide does not guarantee any particular result (e.g., weight loss or a cure). By reading this guide, you acknowledge that there are no guarantees to any specific outcome or results you can expect.

All product names, diet plans, or names used in this guide are for identification purposes only and are the property of their respective owners. The use of these names does not imply endorsement. All other trademarks cited herein are the property of their respective owners.

Where applicable, this guide is not intended to be a substitute for the original work of this diet plan and is, at most, a supplement to the original work for this diet plan and never a direct substitute. This guide is a personal expression of the facts of that diet plan.

Where applicable, persons shown in the cover images are stock photography models and the publisher has obtained the rights to use the images through license agreements with third-party stock image companies.

Table of Contents

Introduction — 8
What Is the Fast Mimicking Diet and How Does It Work? — 11
   Why Follow FMD? — 12
   Difference of FMD to Intermittent Fasting — 14
   The Science Behind FMD — 15
What Makes FMD Unique? — 17
   Benefits of the Fast Mimicking Diet — 18
   Things to Keep in Mind — 20
   Is FMD Right for You? — 21
Understanding the Science Behind FMD — 23
   Autophagy — The Cell's Internal Renewal System — 24
   Ketosis — Adapting to an Alternate Energy Pathway — 25
   IGF-1 Modulation — Adjusting Growth and Repair Priorities — 26
   Interconnected Pathways — A Coordinated Response — 27
   What the Research Shows—and What It Doesn't — 28
Common Myths and Misconceptions About the Fast Mimicking Diet — 30
   Myth 1: FMD keeps the body in fat-burning mode indefinitely — 30
   Myth 2: Post-FMD eating habits don't matter — 31
   Myth 3: FMD is just another form of intermittent fasting — 31
   Myth 4: FMD guarantees deep "cellular detox" — 32
   Myth 5: FMD is safe and effective for everyone — 32
   Myth 6: More cycles mean better results — 33
Psychological and Emotional Aspects of the Fast Mimicking Diet — 35
   Why FMD Feels Mentally Different — 35
   Cravings: A Response to Biology, Emotion, and Environment — 36

Decision Fatigue and Mental Energy	37
Emotional Regulation with Lower Calorie Intake	38
Mindfulness as a Practical Tool	39
Changing the Eating Environment	39
Recognizing Physical Hunger vs. Emotional Urges	40
Accepting the Challenge	42
Preparing for Future Rounds	43
Customizing the Fast Mimicking Diet for Different Goals	**45**
For Weight Loss and Body Composition	45
For Metabolic Health and Biomarker Support	47
For Longevity and Healthy Aging	49
FMD in Real Life: Practical Scenarios, Challenges & Long-Term Integration	**52**
Adapting FMD to Different Lifestyles	52
Common Challenges and Targeted Strategies	54
Integrating FMD into a Yearly Routine	55
Psychological Resilience and Motivation	56
Safety and Professional Guidance	57
FMD for Different Age Groups	**58**
Young Adults (Ages 18–30)	58
Adults in Midlife (Ages 30–55)	61
Older Adults (Ages 60+)	62
Teens and Adolescents (Under Age 18)	64
A Personalized, Age-Informed Approach	65
Foods to Eat and Avoid on the Fast Mimicking Diet	**67**
Foods to Include	68
Foods to Limit or Avoid	71
Hydration & Beverages	72
Supplement Considerations	73
Structuring a Day's Intake	73
After the FMD Cycle	74

The Two-Week Fast Mimicking Diet Plan	**75**
Week 1 – Preparation & Adaptation	75
Week 2 – Core FMD Phase	78
Recovery & Transition (Days 7–8 of Week 2)	80
Key Considerations for Both Weeks	81
Why the Two-Week Structure Works	82
Sample Recipes	**83**
Kale Lentil Bowl	84
Zucchini & Olive Salad	86
Roasted Cauliflower with Tahini Drizzle	87
Sweet Potato & Walnut Mash	88
Spinach Avocado Wrap	89
Cucumber & Avocado Salad	90
Roasted Carrots with Sesame	91
Warm Quinoa & Vegetable Bowl	92
Eggplant with Garlic Tahini Sauce	93
Tomato & Basil Zoodle Bowl	94
Steamed Broccoli with Almond Drizzle	95
Beet & Orange Salad	96
Roasted Brussels Sprouts with Lemon Oil	97
Mediterranean Chickpea Salad	98
Roasted Red Pepper & Almond Dip	99
Spiced Pumpkin Soup	100
Conclusion	**102**
Frequently Asked Questions	**105**
References and Helpful Links	**109**

Introduction

Interest in the biological effects of fasting has grown significantly over the past decade, particularly in relation to metabolic health, cellular stress responses, and the biology of aging. A growing body of research is exploring how the body responds to short-term reductions in calorie and nutrient intake — and how these responses might be leveraged in ways that are both structured and sustainable.

One area of investigation examines whether certain dietary patterns can temporarily engage fasting-related cellular processes, such as nutrient sensing, ketone production, and autophagy, while still allowing some degree of food consumption. Some early studies suggest that carefully timed and nutritionally calibrated approaches may activate similar metabolic pathways to those seen in traditional fasting, though outcomes vary by individual and more research is needed to confirm long-term effects.

This guide offers a detailed overview of one such dietary model — an approach developed through academic research and tested in clinical settings. It is intended for readers seeking to better understand the science, structure, and applications of short-term, food-inclusive dietary strategies that aim to support biological renewal while maintaining safety and nutritional adequacy.

In this guide, we will explore:

- A clear definition of the Fast Mimicking Diet (FMD) and how it differs from other fasting strategies
- Key mechanisms such as autophagy, ketosis, and insulin-like growth factor-1 (IGF-1) modulation
- The role of macronutrient composition in mimicking fasting states
- Example food guidelines, recipes, and a two-week phased plan
- Considerations for safety, individual suitability, and potential benefits

Important: This guide does not make therapeutic claims or promote fasting as a treatment for any condition. It is not a substitute for individualized medical care. FMD is not appropriate for everyone, and individuals with specific health conditions — including those who are pregnant, underweight, managing diabetes, or with a history of disordered eating — should consult a qualified healthcare provider before making dietary changes.

The goal of this guide is to present the available information in a clear, accessible, and medically cautious way. By understanding how the Fast Mimicking Diet works, individuals can make informed decisions about whether it aligns with their nutritional goals, health status, and personal needs.

What Is the Fast Mimicking Diet and How Does It Work?

The Fast Mimicking Diet (FMD) is a structured approach to eating that *may mimic some of the biological effects of fasting* without requiring complete food deprivation. It was developed from research on how the body responds to short-term nutrient restriction, particularly in relation to cellular maintenance, energy balance, and aging.

Instead of complete food abstinence, FMD uses a carefully controlled combination of *reduced total calories* and specific macronutrient ratios. The goal is to *modulate nutrient-sensing pathways*, including insulin and IGF-1, which are involved in growth and cellular maintenance. Protein and certain amino acids are kept low, while complex carbohydrates and healthy fats are emphasized. As a result, the body may shift toward increased fat metabolism and the production of ketones, which *may support processes like autophagy*, the body's natural cellular repair mechanism.

Dr. Valter Longo, a cell biologist, played a pivotal role in developing FMD, having studied the relationship between nutrient patterns, fasting signals, and longevity. His research showed that precise modulation of calories and nutrients over a five-day period could trigger metabolic responses similar to those seen in complete fasting.

FMD is practiced in cycles, with normal eating typically resuming after each fasting-mimicking phase. These cycles create brief periods of metabolic stress followed by recovery, which *may help maintain cellular function*. While biomarkers like IGF-1, glucose, and ketones may change during FMD, individual responses vary, and long-term effects are still being researched. This approach is not intended as a therapeutic diet but offers a framework based on *available research* for those interested in exploring fasting's biological principles in a sustainable way.

Why Follow FMD?

Interest in the Fast Mimicking Diet (FMD) has grown in parallel with increased attention to metabolic health, longevity research, and sustainable approaches to calorie reduction. Many are drawn to the concept because it offers a defined, time-limited structure—a short period of modified eating—rather than continuous or indefinite restrictions. This can make it seem more manageable than traditional fasting or long-term dieting.

At its core, FMD is designed to create a temporary shift in metabolic activity. By adjusting calorie intake and macronutrient composition for a set period, it may influence certain measurable markers — such as blood glucose, ketones, and IGF-1 — that researchers study for their potential roles in energy regulation, cellular maintenance, and stress adaptation. The aim is to encourage these short-term changes while still providing some nourishment. This approach may help some individuals experience greater focus and a calmer mood compared with complete fasting, though responses can vary widely.

Another benefit is the cyclical nature of FMD. Since it is typically practiced in short intervals—often five days at a time—it can be more easily integrated into a broader lifestyle without requiring constant attention to food choices. This structured approach offers flexibility: there is a clear beginning and end, which can help make the process feel more manageable.

From a practical standpoint, FMD encourages a plant-based, minimally processed diet during the fasting-mimicking phase, which aligns with dietary patterns linked to positive health outcomes in various studies. Many people also report that the short duration of the diet helps them reflect on their eating habits and reintroduce foods more consciously afterward.

While FMD is not intended to replace medical care, its potential benefits are best viewed as part of a balanced, overall lifestyle. It is important to consult with a healthcare provider who can assess whether FMD aligns with your health goals and needs, especially since it may not be suitable for everyone.

Difference of FMD to Intermittent Fasting

While both the Fast Mimicking Diet (FMD) and Intermittent Fasting (IF) are forms of short-term dietary restriction, they use different methods to achieve their effects. FMD focuses on structured food intake over several days, while IF emphasizes timing of eating and fasting periods within each day or week. The table below highlights key differences to help clarify how each approach works.

Table: Features between FMD and Intermittent Fasting

Feature	Fast Mimicking Diet (FMD)	Intermittent Fasting (IF)
Primary Focus	Nutrient composition over several days	Timing of food intake within 24-hour cycles
Duration	5 consecutive days (typical protocol)	Daily (e.g., 16:8), or alternating fasting/eating days
Food Intake	Limited calories (~700–1100/day), structured macros	Minimal or no calories during fasting periods
Macronutrient Design	Low protein, low carbs, moderate-to-high healthy fats	No specific macronutrient focus
Metabolic Goal	Mimic prolonged fasting response	Create short fasting windows to support metabolic shifts
Common Responses	Ketosis, IGF-1 reduction, fat	Ketosis (in longer fasts), glucose

	metabolism	regulation
Protocol Frequency	Typically once per month or seasonally	Often practiced several times per week or daily
Eating Schedule	Set meal plan over 5 days	Eating limited to specific windows (e.g., 12pm–8pm)
Typical Use Case	Short-term metabolic reset, structured intervention	Ongoing eating pattern, flexible integration
Suitability	Requires planning; not suitable for all individuals	May be easier to adopt gradually, though not for everyone

Both strategies may support metabolic flexibility in different ways. Choosing between them depends on personal preferences, health goals, and whether a time-based or nutrient-based structure feels more sustainable.

The Science Behind FMD

The Fast Mimicking Diet (FMD) works by adjusting calorie intake and macronutrient composition in ways that may temporarily trigger some of the same nutrient-sensing pathways observed during fasting. Studies have shown associations between FMD cycles and short-term shifts in several measurable markers, including blood glucose, ketones, and insulin-like growth factor 1 (IGF-1).

In research settings, participants often experience a modest decrease in fasting glucose and insulin levels during the fasting-mimicking phase. As carbohydrate availability drops, the body may increase its reliance on fat for fuel, producing small amounts of ketones. These molecules are an alternative energy source and have been studied for potential roles in metabolic flexibility and cellular resilience.

Another observed change is a temporary reduction in IGF-1, a hormone involved in cell growth and metabolism. Lower levels are associated in some studies with reduced growth signaling, which may create a biological environment more favorable to maintenance and repair.

These responses are not guaranteed and can vary by individual, depending on baseline health, diet between cycles, and other lifestyle factors. Most human trials to date have been small and short in duration, so long-term implications remain uncertain.

While the science is still developing, FMD offers a structured framework for exploring fasting-related biology without complete food abstinence. For a detailed look at specific mechanisms — including autophagy, ketosis, and IGF-1 modulation — see **Understanding the Science Behind FMD**.

What Makes FMD Unique?

The Fast Mimicking Diet is distinct in its ability to trigger fasting-like responses while still allowing limited food intake. This is achieved through a deliberate macronutrient structure — typically low in protein, moderate in healthy fats, and relatively low in carbohydrates. By reducing overall calorie intake and adjusting nutrient ratios, FMD is designed to avoid activating nutrient-sensing pathways that normally signal the body to stay in a "fed" state.

Unlike traditional water-only fasts, which can be physically and emotionally challenging, FMD includes food in a way that may reduce hunger, fatigue, and mood fluctuations. This can make it easier for many people to complete multi-day cycles while maintaining basic daily routines.

Because the body still receives some fuel, FMD may help sustain mental focus and emotional stability during the fasting-mimicking phase. This blend of physiological benefit and greater ease of use makes it a more accessible option for those exploring structured fasting in a science-informed, short-term format.

Benefits of the Fast Mimicking Diet

(For underlying mechanisms and evidence limitations, see The Science Behind FMD, p. X.)

Current research — though still limited in size and duration — suggests several areas where FMD may influence biological processes associated with fasting. These include:

1. **Has been associated in limited studies with potential cellular stress resilience**

   Short, structured reductions in calories and protein have been linked in some studies to nutrient-sensing pathways involved in maintenance and repair. Early findings in both animals and humans suggest these shifts may be part of the body's adaptation to nutrient changes. Because results vary, they should be considered potential effects rather than guaranteed outcomes.

2. **Has Been Associated With Temporary IGF-1 Reductions**

   IGF-1 (insulin-like growth factor 1) helps regulate growth and cell signaling. Elevated levels have been linked to increased cell proliferation. In some participants, short-term FMD cycles have been associated with temporary reductions in IGF-1, which may influence growth-related pathways.

3. **May Support Shifts in Fat Metabolism and Waist Measurements**

   In certain clinical studies, participants experienced temporary reductions in abdominal fat and body weight, alongside indications of greater fat-to-energy conversion. These effects were observed in some individuals without ongoing calorie restriction and may reflect short-term improvements in metabolic flexibility. Results vary based on factors such as baseline health, eating patterns between cycles, and activity levels.

4. **Could Influence Markers of Inflammation and Glucose Regulation**

   Preliminary human research suggests FMD may be associated with modest improvements in fasting glucose, insulin, and certain inflammatory markers. These shifts are not universal and often return toward baseline after resuming normal eating.

5. **May Offer a More Sustainable Fasting Approach**

   Because it includes food, FMD may be easier for some people to repeat compared to full fasting. This structure can help reduce the common discomforts of fasting while still engaging certain metabolic pathways.

Things to Keep in Mind

The Fast Mimicking Diet (FMD) is a short, structured form of reduced-calorie eating that adjusts macronutrient ratios to create fasting-like effects. Even with food included, it places the body in a controlled, low-energy state that can influence mood, energy, and metabolic processes.

FMD is ***not appropriate*** for:

- Anyone who is underweight (BMI below the healthy range)
- Pregnant or breastfeeding individuals
- People under 18
- Those with a history of disordered eating or restrictive dieting
- Individuals with type 1 diabetes, insulin use, or other glucose-lowering medications without medical supervision
- People recovering from surgery, illness, or managing chronic conditions that require consistent caloric intake
- Those with frailty, certain thyroid, adrenal, or gastrointestinal conditions, or anyone taking prescription medication without clearance from a healthcare provider

Short-term effects can include fatigue, irritability, digestive changes, or sleep disturbances, which generally resolve once normal eating resumes. To determine suitability and avoid complications, consult a qualified healthcare provider before starting, especially if you have medical conditions, take prescription drugs, or fall into a higher-risk group.

Is FMD Right for You?

FMD can shift certain metabolic markers in the short term, but it involves significant dietary change and is not suitable for everyone. A healthcare professional should assess your health, medication use, and daily energy demands before you begin.

Seek professional guidance if you:

- Have a BMI under 18.5
- Are pregnant, breastfeeding, or trying to conceive
- Are younger than 18 or older than 70
- Have diabetes, kidney disease, cancer, or other major medical conditions
- Are recovering from illness, injury, or surgery
- Take medication for blood sugar, blood pressure, or other chronic conditions
- Experience dizziness, fainting, or unusual fatigue with reduced food intake
- Have a history of eating disorders or high-restriction diets
- Perform physically demanding work or intense exercise

- Are under significant stress or find routine changes difficult

FMD is best suited to generally healthy adults without medical restrictions. It should be adapted to your personal health history, needs, and long-term goals.

Understanding the Science Behind FMD

The Fast Mimicking Diet has gained attention for its ability to simulate some of the same biological responses seen during traditional fasting, while still allowing limited food intake. At first glance, the concept seems straightforward: reduce calories for a few days, adjust macronutrient ratios, and let the body respond. Yet the changes that occur beneath the surface involve intricate signaling networks and adaptive responses shaped by human evolution.

When the body senses a temporary reduction in energy and protein availability, it can shift priorities away from growth and reproduction and toward maintenance, repair, and conservation of resources. Researchers studying FMD have identified several processes that appear to play a central role in this shift: **autophagy**, **ketosis**, and ***IGF-1 modulation***. These pathways are not isolated "switches" — they overlap, influence each other, and respond to multiple inputs at once, including nutrient levels, hormone signals, and energy demand.

Autophagy — The Cell's Internal Renewal System

Autophagy, literally "self-eating," is the body's built-in recycling and quality-control program. Damaged proteins, malfunctioning mitochondria, and other worn-out cellular components are broken down, and the raw materials are reused to sustain essential functions. It's as though every cell has a maintenance crew that dismantles old parts, salvages what can be used, and discards what no longer serves a purpose.

In animal research, periods of calorie or nutrient restriction have been shown to enhance autophagy in multiple tissues, including the brain, liver, and skeletal muscle. This process is thought to help cells adapt to stress by prioritizing repair over expansion.

In humans, direct evidence is harder to obtain, as autophagy cannot be easily measured in living tissue. Instead, researchers use indirect indicators — for example, reductions in insulin and circulating amino acids, combined with increases in ketone production — to infer when conditions may favor autophagic activity.

Studies have found that FMD-style eating, which combines low calorie intake with reduced protein, can produce these same nutrient-sensing signals in some individuals. However, the degree and consistency of autophagy activation in humans remain open questions, and more large-scale research is needed to clarify its magnitude and duration.

Ketosis — Adapting to an Alternate Energy Pathway

Ketosis is a metabolic state in which the body shifts from using glucose as its primary fuel to relying on fat stores. When carbohydrates become scarce and insulin levels fall, the liver converts fatty acids into molecules called ketones, which can serve as an efficient energy source for the brain, muscles, and other tissues.

This is not a new "biohack" — it is a deeply rooted survival strategy that allowed humans to function for days or weeks when food was scarce. In the context of FMD, mild ketosis often emerges by the second or third day, as carbohydrate availability drops and healthy fats from plant sources supply steady energy.

Some studies have observed associations between short-term, mild ketosis during FMD and shifts in mitochondrial function, energy regulation, and markers of cellular stress resilience. Importantly, ketosis is not inherently superior to glucose metabolism. Rather, it represents an alternate mode of operation that the body can move in and out of, depending on energy availability. In FMD, this temporary fuel shift is one part of a broader adaptive package, not the sole goal.

IGF-1 Modulation — Adjusting Growth and Repair Priorities

Insulin-like growth factor 1 (IGF-1) is a hormone that plays a vital role in tissue growth, repair, and metabolic signaling. While essential for development and healing, sustained high IGF-1 levels have been linked in some studies to increased rates of cell proliferation — a process that, over a lifetime, may contribute to aging-related changes.

FMD cycles have been associated in research with short-lived reductions in IGF-1, often accompanied by lower glucose and insulin levels. These hormonal changes may shift the body's focus from building new tissue toward maintaining and repairing what already exists. This is one reason FMD is sometimes discussed in longevity research, where the balance between growth and preservation is considered central to healthy aging.

However, IGF-1 is not inherently harmful. Extremely low levels can impair muscle retention, wound healing, and immune response. The cyclical nature of FMD — where IGF-1 dips during the fasting-mimicking phase and then rebounds with normal eating — may help capture some of the potential benefits of reduced growth signaling without long-term suppression.

Interconnected Pathways — A Coordinated Response

These three processes influence and reinforce each other through a network of nutrient-sensing systems. For example:

- Lower protein intake during FMD can downregulate mTOR signaling, a key regulator of growth, while simultaneously favoring conditions that support autophagy.
- The onset of ketosis often parallels reductions in insulin and glucose, which can further affect IGF-1 signaling.
- Energy-regulating enzymes such as AMPK and proteins like sirtuins respond to these nutrient shifts, with potential downstream effects on inflammation, mitochondrial efficiency, and stress adaptation.

This web of interactions reflects the body's capacity to reprioritize during times of scarcity. FMD leverages this adaptation in a time-limited, structured format, allowing for a temporary "maintenance mode" without requiring complete fasting.

While these mechanisms are well documented in animal studies and supported by emerging human research, the translation to long-term health outcomes is still being explored. Individual responses vary widely, shaped by factors such as age, metabolic health, diet outside of FMD cycles, and genetic predisposition.

What the Research Shows—and What It Doesn't

Much of what we know about FMD's biological effects comes from a mix of preclinical research, small human trials, and observational studies. In animal models, cycles of fasting or FMD have been associated with changes in body composition, metabolic markers, immune modulation, and extended lifespan. In humans, trials have documented shifts in:

- Glucose and insulin sensitivity
- Ketone production
- IGF-1 levels
- C-reactive protein (CRP), a marker of inflammation
- Triglyceride levels and other lipids

Still, these findings must be interpreted carefully. The magnitude of change varies by individual, and many studies are short in duration or limited in scope. FMD is not a guaranteed method for achieving long-term outcomes—and its effects likely depend on context, consistency, and overall health status.

FMD operates on the body's natural ability to adapt under nutrient stress. It may activate pathways linked to repair, metabolic balance, and longevity—but these shifts are subtle, temporary, and context-specific. The science behind FMD is promising, but still evolving, and it's essential to view it not as a magic bullet, but as one possible tool in a broader health strategy.

When practiced appropriately—and with professional guidance where needed—FMD can offer a glimpse into how the body recalibrates when given structured rest from the constant influx of nutrients. But like any health practice, its value lies in how it fits into the individual's unique biology, goals, and lifestyle.

Common Myths and Misconceptions About the Fast Mimicking Diet

Despite growing awareness of the Fast Mimicking Diet (FMD), misconceptions still circulate—some based on outdated science, others on overhyped marketing. This chapter clarifies common myths using current research, helping readers approach FMD with balanced expectations and informed judgment.

Myth 1: FMD keeps the body in fat-burning mode indefinitely

Some believe that completing an FMD cycle triggers a lasting shift into fat metabolism. In reality, while the diet can temporarily raise fat oxidation and ketone production—often by Day 2 or 3—these changes are short-lived. Once normal calorie and carbohydrate intake resumes, glucose returns as the primary energy source. Current studies show no evidence that a single cycle creates a permanent metabolic change without ongoing dietary strategies.

Safety note: Individual fat-burning results vary and depend on factors such as baseline diet, activity level, and overall health.

Myth 2: Post-FMD eating habits don't matter

A common misconception is that after FMD, the body can tolerate unrestricted eating—including high-sugar or ultra-processed foods—without undoing the benefits. In fact, the period immediately after a cycle is one in which the body is especially responsive to nutrient signals. In clinical trials, participants resumed balanced, whole-food diets after FMD, not indulgent eating. How someone eats in the days following a cycle influences whether metabolic markers stabilize, improve, or regress.

Practical takeaway: Think of FMD as part of a broader eating pattern, not a free pass to abandon nutrition principles.

Myth 3: FMD is just another form of intermittent fasting

While both approaches involve periods of lower calorie intake, they differ in structure and physiological emphasis. Intermittent fasting typically limits eating to certain hours each day or alternates fasting and eating days. FMD, in contrast, focuses on what and how much you eat over several consecutive days, with defined macronutrient targets. Research suggests the two strategies can influence markers like IGF-1 and inflammation differently, though both have been linked to metabolic shifts.

Context to keep in mind: Neither method is universally better. The right choice depends on health status, goals, and personal preference.

Myth 4: FMD guarantees deep "cellular detox"

Some promotional claims suggest FMD ensures intense cellular cleansing or complete autophagy. Autophagy is a natural recycling process that may increase during nutrient restriction, but measuring it directly in humans is challenging. Most of what's known comes from animal studies, where nutrient stress enhanced autophagy in various tissues. In people, indirect markers—such as lower insulin or amino acid levels—indicate conditions that may support the process, but effects vary.

Important note: FMD should not be promoted as a detox program. Any discussion of autophagy needs to be framed as a potential, not guaranteed, response.

Myth 5: FMD is safe and effective for everyone

Because FMD is short-term and includes food, it can be mistaken for a universally safe option. In reality, some groups face higher risks from calorie restriction—even in modified forms. People who are underweight, pregnant, breastfeeding, under 18, or managing medical conditions such as diabetes, cardiovascular disease, or eating disorders may experience negative effects from the diet.

Clinical research on FMD has largely focused on generally healthy adults or those with specific metabolic risk factors, and vulnerable populations are typically excluded. Where benefits have been observed, they have occurred under medical supervision.

Key takeaway: FMD is not a one-size-fits-all approach. Anyone with a medical condition, taking prescription medication, or belonging to a higher-risk group should only attempt it with professional guidance.

Myth 6: More cycles mean better results

Some assume that stacking FMD cycles back-to-back or repeating them frequently will amplify results such as fat loss, increased energy, or cellular renewal. However, the body needs recovery time between periods of nutrient stress. Overdoing fasting-mimicking cycles can lead to fatigue, nutrient gaps, and hormonal imbalances.

Most human studies have tested FMD once a month for 3–4 months, spacing cycles to allow normal eating in between. These intervals help maintain nutritional adequacy and overall well-being. There is no long-term evidence supporting frequent or continuous use without breaks.

Key takeaway: More is not always better. The safest frequency depends on individual health status, recovery capacity, and professional recommendations.

Psychological and Emotional Aspects of the Fast Mimicking Diet

The Fast Mimicking Diet (FMD) is designed to prompt metabolic changes without requiring complete abstinence from food. Even in a short-term plan, a shift in calorie intake affects more than physical health. Hunger sensations, mood changes, and altered routines can influence how the mind processes decisions and emotions.

Understanding these mental and emotional patterns before beginning FMD helps set realistic expectations. When you know that cravings, irritability, or restlessness are common, they feel less like a sign that the plan is failing and more like a natural stage in the process. This awareness allows you to approach the experience with preparation instead of surprise.

Why FMD Feels Mentally Different

The human brain is quick to detect changes in energy supply. When calorie intake decreases, the body releases signals that encourage eating. Hormones such as ghrelin, which stimulates appetite, often increase, while leptin, which signals satiety, may decrease. These changes make food seem more appealing, sometimes in ways that feel unusually strong.

The mental adjustment often goes beyond hunger alone. Many people experience a disruption of daily patterns. Breakfast meetings, coffee breaks, or evening snacks are more than calorie sources; they are cues that shape daily rhythm. Altering or removing them can lead to a sense of restlessness or loss. The first few days of FMD are when these feelings are most noticeable. As the body adapts, the new structure begins to feel more familiar.

Cravings: A Response to Biology, Emotion, and Environment

Cravings during FMD are common, and they often result from a mix of physical and psychological factors.

Biological influences

Reduced calorie intake can heighten the brain's reward sensitivity, making high-calorie foods seem more enticing. This change is a normal neurological response to reduced energy availability.

Emotional triggers

Stress, boredom, and anxiety often increase the desire for comfort foods. These cravings may occur even when the body has enough fuel, because the urge is driven by emotion rather than energy needs.

Environmental cues

Visual, auditory, and olfactory cues can spark cravings. Walking past a bakery, smelling food being prepared, or seeing someone eat can create a sudden desire to eat, even if you were not thinking about food moments earlier.

Recognizing the role of these influences helps you prepare for them. Awareness makes it easier to respond deliberately instead of reacting automatically.

Decision Fatigue and Mental Energy

Repeated acts of self-control can be mentally exhausting. On FMD, this often appears as a constant series of small food-related decisions: "Should I eat now? Is this within the plan? Would it be better to wait?" Over time, the effort involved in making these choices can feel depleting.

Psychologists call this *decision fatigue*. It affects many areas of life, not only eating habits. People often find it harder to stick to a plan in the evening after a full day of choices and problem-solving.

Ways to reduce decision fatigue

- Plan meals and snacks in advance to remove uncertainty.
- Keep FMD-friendly foods accessible and store other foods out of immediate reach.

- Structure your day so that high-craving periods are occupied with non-food activities such as light movement, short walks, or focused work.

The less time spent debating food choices, the more mental energy is available for other tasks.

Emotional Regulation with Lower Calorie Intake

Changes in calorie intake can influence mood through both physical and emotional pathways. Fluctuations in blood sugar may cause temporary irritability, fatigue, or trouble concentrating. Limiting food variety or quantity can also bring a feeling of deprivation, particularly if eating is tied to comfort or social connection.

Common emotional changes during FMD

- Irritability or shorter temper
- Mild anxiety or unease
- Reduced motivation for tasks not related to food
- Increased focus on thoughts about eating

These effects tend to be strongest during the first two days of the plan. As the body adjusts to using stored energy, many people notice their mood stabilizing.

Mindfulness as a Practical Tool

Mindfulness is the practice of paying attention to the present moment without rushing to react. During FMD, mindfulness can help you notice a craving, pause, and choose a response instead of acting on the first impulse.

Steps for using mindfulness during FMD

1. *Notice the sensation*. Identify whether it feels like an empty stomach, a dry mouth, or a thought about a specific food.
2. *Acknowledge without judgment*. Accept that cravings are part of the process.
3. *Pause for a few deep breaths*. This creates space between the feeling and the action.
4. *Choose intentionally*. Decide whether to have a planned food, drink water, or focus on another activity.

Over time, this skill strengthens self-awareness and supports steadier emotional responses.

Changing the Eating Environment

Eating patterns are often shaped by environmental triggers. When a person consistently eats in a certain context, that context becomes a cue for hunger. If you usually snack while watching television, turning on the television may automatically make you think about food.

Identifying common triggers
- Watching specific shows or scrolling through social media that features food
- Passing familiar food locations, such as office break rooms
- Sitting at the dining table at times you used to eat a larger meal

Adjusting triggers during FMD
- Change the physical location of common activities.
- Shift the timing of breaks to avoid overlap with usual snack periods.
- Replace food-related rituals with new ones, such as making herbal tea or stretching.

These changes reduce the number of moments when you must resist temptation.

Recognizing Physical Hunger vs. Emotional Urges

One of the most useful skills to develop during the Fast Mimicking Diet is the ability to separate physical hunger from urges driven by emotion or habit. When food intake is reduced, these two sensations often become easier to tell apart.

Physical hunger is the body's genuine signal that it needs energy. It usually develops gradually, starting with a light sense of emptiness in the stomach or a gentle rumble. If food is not eaten, the sensations may grow stronger and may be accompanied by lower energy, reduced focus, or mild irritability. Physical hunger can generally be satisfied by a wide variety of foods because the body is seeking fuel, not a specific flavor.

Emotional urges to eat arise more abruptly. They are often linked to specific foods and occur in response to a feeling, situation, or cue — such as stress, boredom, celebration, or the sight or smell of food. In these cases, eating serves as comfort, distraction, or reward rather than replenishment of energy stores.

Why the Difference Matters

During FMD, understanding this distinction helps maintain the structure of the plan and encourages more mindful eating. Beyond the diet itself, the skill of identifying hunger type supports long-term eating awareness and reduces unnecessary or impulsive food choices.

A Three-Step Self-Check Before Eating

1. **Rate your hunger on a 1–10 scale**

    A rating of 1 represents extreme hunger, while 10 indicates feeling uncomfortably full. Ratings below 4 often suggest the body may not truly need fuel and the urge could be emotional.

2. **Identify what happened just before the craving**

    Notice whether a specific event, feeling, or environmental cue triggered the desire to eat.

3. **Wait ten minutes and focus on another activity**

    Use the time to do something unrelated to food, such as light movement or a simple task. If the craving fades or changes, it is likely emotional. If it persists, it may indicate physical hunger.

With repetition, this process becomes faster and more intuitive. Over time, it helps create a clearer sense of what the body needs versus what the mind wants, making it easier to respond appropriately in the moment.

Accepting the Challenge

Adjusting to the Fast Mimicking Diet can bring moments of discomfort. Hunger may feel stronger than expected, mood may shift more quickly, and daily routines may feel unsettled. These experiences are not signs that the plan is unsuitable; they are normal reactions to a change in eating pattern and calorie intake.

Recognizing that these responses are temporary can make them easier to manage. Many people find that the most challenging sensations occur in the first one or two days and then begin to level out as the body adapts. This knowledge can help reduce frustration and encourage persistence through the initial adjustment period.

Some participants use these moments as opportunities for observation. Paying attention to when hunger strikes most strongly, how mood changes in relation to eating, and which situations spark cravings can uncover valuable information about personal eating patterns. This insight often carries over into daily life after the FMD cycle ends, supporting more thoughtful food choices and greater self-awareness.

Preparing for Future Rounds

For those planning to follow FMD more than once, the first experience can serve as a useful reference point for future success. Treat it as a trial run that offers information about what works well and what needs adjustment.

Keeping a short record during the cycle can make this process easier. Consider noting:

- Times of day when cravings were most noticeable
- Emotional states that tended to trigger eating urges
- Non-food strategies that provided the most relief or distraction

Reviewing these notes before the next round allows for targeted preparation. You can plan meals or activities to address high-craving periods, anticipate emotional triggers, and repeat strategies that proved effective. This preparation not only increases confidence but also helps reduce the mental effort required during subsequent cycles.

When to Seek Help

If mood changes or cravings feel unmanageable, or if the plan stirs up past struggles with restrictive eating, it is important to pause and speak with a healthcare provider. Support from a registered dietitian or therapist can help ensure the approach is both safe and sustainable.

Cravings during the Fast Mimicking Diet can stem from a combination of biological, emotional, and environmental influences. Planning ahead and reducing the number of food-related decisions may help preserve mental energy for some individuals throughout the process. Mindfulness techniques and small changes to the eating environment often make it easier to manage both hunger and emotional strain.

Developing the ability to recognize the difference between physical hunger and emotional urges is a valuable skill that can extend beyond the diet itself. Challenges are a normal part of adapting to a new eating pattern, and approaching them with preparation and self-awareness can make them more manageable.

Customizing the Fast Mimicking Diet for Different Goals

The Fast Mimicking Diet (FMD) offers a structured approach to temporary caloric restriction while maintaining some food intake, making it adaptable for various wellness goals. While the core principles remain the same—low-calorie, low-protein, plant-forward meals over a short period—individuals may approach the diet with different intentions.

Whether the goal is reshaping body composition, supporting metabolic markers, or exploring longevity research, customization should be thoughtful, medically guided, and aligned with realistic expectations.

For Weight Loss and Body Composition

Weight loss is a common motivator for individuals exploring FMD, but results can vary. The approach is best considered a structured metabolic intervention rather than a guaranteed or rapid fat-loss method.

What the Research Shows

Several studies, including clinical trials in adults, have found that periodic use of an FMD protocol has been observed in some research to coincide with modest reductions in total body fat, particularly visceral fat, in certain participants. In some small research studies, certain participants experienced temporary reductions in waist circumference and fat mass over several cycles, though results varied and not all participants saw these changes.

These changes often occurred without major losses in lean body mass—likely due to the low but strategic inclusion of carbohydrates and fats during the fasting window.

Still, these outcomes can vary widely. Some individuals may not observe significant changes on the scale, particularly if they're already lean or metabolically healthy. That's why body weight alone is a limited metric.

Shifting the Focus: Metrics That Matter

When customizing FMD for weight-related goals, it may be more helpful to track markers beyond pounds lost. Some individuals report:

- A decrease in waist circumference
- Greater ease maintaining portion control post-cycle
- Improvements in fasting glucose or triglyceride levels
- Enhanced mood stability or reduced cravings
- Less bloating and digestive heaviness

Tracking body composition (via DEXA scans or bioimpedance devices), energy levels, sleep quality, and inflammation markers such as CRP (C-reactive protein) may provide a more complete picture than the scale alone.

Frequency and Timing Considerations

Weight-related outcomes may be more evident after multiple cycles. Some protocols suggest monthly or bi-monthly use for a few months, depending on individual baseline metrics. However, it's essential not to treat FMD as a recurring diet without breaks or oversight. Fatigue, micronutrient insufficiency, and potential hormonal effects can arise with overly frequent cycles.

A common approach is to start with one cycle, monitor outcomes with your healthcare provider, then reassess whether additional rounds are appropriate. Individuals with significant weight to lose may consider pairing FMD with sustainable eating patterns between cycles rather than relying on it as a standalone strategy.

For Metabolic Health and Biomarker Support

Some individuals turn to FMD with the goal of supporting markers related to chronic disease risk—such as blood sugar, cholesterol, and inflammatory status. While the Fast Mimicking Diet is not a treatment or cure for any condition, early research suggests it may influence internal signals related to metabolic function.

A Metabolic "Reset" Approach

FMD induces a low-energy, low-protein state that nudges the body into nutrient-sensing shifts typically seen in water-only fasting—without requiring complete food abstinence. During these phases, some studies have shown changes in:

- Fasting glucose and insulin sensitivity
- Ketone levels (mild, due to fat intake)
- IGF-1 (Insulin-like Growth Factor 1)
- Inflammatory cytokines
- Triglycerides and LDL particles

These shifts are often temporary and can vary in degree. Some researchers hypothesize that when repeated in cycles, these fluctuations may help influence or adjust how the body responds to food, stress, and metabolic stressors. However, the magnitude and durability of these changes are still under investigation.

Emerging Links with Chronic Disease Markers

Emerging research suggests that FMD has been studied for potential associations with biomarkers linked to metabolic syndrome, prediabetes, or cardiovascular risk in specific populations in certain populations.

For example, a 2017 randomized trial published in Science Translational Medicine observed reductions in fasting glucose, blood pressure, and abdominal fat among individuals who followed multiple FMD cycles over three months. These changes were more pronounced in participants with higher baseline risk.

It's worth noting, however, that these results are associative, not causative. The effects were seen in small, controlled cohorts and should not be generalized as prescriptive for managing medical conditions.

Caution for Those with Diagnosed Conditions

FMD is not appropriate for individuals on glucose-lowering medications, those with insulin-dependent diabetes, or anyone managing a chronic condition without clinical supervision. Caloric restriction—even when partial—can impact medication timing, blood sugar dynamics, and electrolyte balance.

Anyone interested in using FMD as a way to monitor or influence metabolic biomarkers should first work with a qualified health professional to ensure compatibility with their current regimen.

For Longevity and Healthy Aging

Interest in fasting and caloric restriction has surged among those exploring lifestyle strategies for longevity. The appeal of FMD for this group lies in its structured, cyclical nature—offering a repeatable "reset" without the burden of constant restriction.

The Longevity Hypothesis

In laboratory studies involving animals and cellular models, periodic fasting has been observed in research to correlate with changes in signaling pathways that influence cell growth, inflammation, and energy metabolism. One of the most studied pathways involves IGF-1, a growth factor linked to aging and cellular turnover. Lowering IGF-1 through short-term dietary interventions may influence processes like autophagy (cellular cleanup) and stress resistance.

In humans, the evidence is still evolving. Some early trials suggest that FMD cycles may temporarily reduce IGF-1 levels and increase markers of cellular stress adaptation. However, the connection between these shifts and long-term health outcomes remains theoretical at this stage.

Individualized Longevity Strategies

When used for healthy aging, FMD is often positioned as one part of a broader routine that includes:

- Regular movement and strength training
- Plant-forward, nutrient-dense eating patterns
- Stress reduction techniques
- Adequate sleep and circadian rhythm support

Rather than relying solely on FMD as a longevity tool, many longevity-focused individuals use it to complement these practices. One cycle every few months may be sufficient, depending on age, baseline health, and tolerance.

Safety Considerations Across All Goals

Regardless of your reason for trying FMD, medical oversight is essential—especially if any of the following apply:

- You are underweight or have a history of disordered eating
- You take medications for blood pressure, blood sugar, or cholesterol
- You're pregnant, breastfeeding, or planning conception
- You're managing a chronic condition or undergoing medical treatment
- You have a low BMI, frailty, or are over 70

FMD may not be appropriate in these contexts, or it may require modified supervision and personalized adjustments. Customizing the approach does not mean abandoning safety guardrails.

FMD in Real Life: Practical Scenarios, Challenges & Long-Term Integration

The Fast Mimicking Diet (FMD) can sound straightforward on paper: five days of adjusted calories and macronutrients, followed by a return to regular eating. In practice, daily routines, work commitments, travel plans, and personal preferences all shape how the plan unfolds. This chapter explores how to adapt FMD to different lifestyles, anticipate common hurdles, and weave it into a broader health strategy without letting it become disruptive or overly rigid.

Adapting FMD to Different Lifestyles

Busy Professionals

Those with long workdays or unpredictable schedules often benefit from planning meals in advance. Packing lunches, portioning snacks, and having ready-to-eat vegetable dishes or broth can reduce the temptation to grab higher-calorie convenience foods. If work involves back-to-back meetings, liquid options like vegetable soups or blended vegetable drinks can be consumed quickly without skipping nourishment.

Parents and Caregivers

Preparing separate meals for the household can be one of the biggest obstacles. The simplest approach is to make shared dishes that fit the FMD structure—roasted vegetables, salads with olive oil, or soups—while adding protein or grains for other family members. Eating together without feeling like an outsider helps maintain social connection during the cycle.

Active Individuals

Those accustomed to regular workouts may need to scale intensity to match reduced fuel availability. Light strength work, mobility exercises, or restorative yoga can keep movement habits intact while avoiding excessive strain. Scheduling high-output training for the week after FMD can take advantage of the re-feeding period for muscle repair.

Remote Workers

Working from home provides easy access to the kitchen—a benefit and a challenge. Structuring the day with defined eating windows and keeping FMD-friendly meals pre-portioned helps prevent unplanned snacking. Setting a designated "meal area" can also reduce grazing prompted by proximity to food.

Common Challenges and Targeted Strategies

Social Situations

Invitations to eat out can fall during the five-day window. Options include:

- Scheduling FMD for a quieter week with fewer social events.
- Choosing restaurants with vegetable-forward menus where dishes can be adapted.
- Ordering small portions and focusing on low-protein, plant-based sides.

Travel

Airport food courts, hotel dining, and unfamiliar grocery stores can make adherence tricky. Strategies include packing a small supply of nuts, single-serve olive oil packets, and herbal tea bags, and locating nearby markets in advance. Soups, salads, and steamed vegetables are available in many locations with minimal modification.

Hunger and Cravings

For many, Days 2 and 3 bring the strongest appetite signals. Distraction works better than constant suppression—brief walks, phone calls, or non-food hobbies help shift attention. Warm beverages, particularly broth or herbal tea, can provide a sense of fullness without breaking the nutrient balance.

Energy Dips

Gentle pacing throughout the day preserves stamina. Prioritizing demanding mental or physical tasks for morning hours, when energy is often steadier, can reduce frustration. Midday rest periods, even short ones, help manage the natural ebb in alertness.

Integrating FMD into a Yearly Routine

FMD can function as a periodic "reset" without becoming a dominant eating pattern. The frequency should reflect personal tolerance, goals, and recovery capacity.

Quarterly Approach

Completing one cycle every three months can support a rhythm that feels intentional without pushing the body into prolonged nutrient stress.

Seasonal Approach

Some people prefer to align cycles with seasonal transitions—spring cleaning for the body, an autumn recalibration before winter, or a mid-summer lightening period.

Combined with Other Patterns

Between cycles, the focus returns to nutrient sufficiency. Many integrate a plant-forward, Mediterranean-style approach, or maintain light time-restricted eating without strict calorie caps. This balance allows the benefits of short-term fasting signals while supporting ongoing nourishment.

Psychological Resilience and Motivation

Short-term dietary shifts are as much mental as physical. Approaching FMD with a clear reason—whether curiosity about metabolic responses, desire to recalibrate eating habits, or interest in longevity science—can strengthen adherence.

Tracking the Experience

Noting energy levels, digestion, mood, and sleep quality creates a more complete picture than relying on weight alone. Reviewing these notes before each new cycle helps refine the process.

Avoiding Perfection Pressure

A missed portion or timing slip does not erase the potential value of the cycle. The goal is consistency across the five days, not flawless execution.

Adjusting Over Time

FMD is not static. Energy demands, stress levels, and health status shift, and the diet should be responsive to those changes.

- During high-stress months, reducing frequency or delaying a cycle can prevent compounding strain.

- After illness or injury, recovery should take priority before resuming calorie restriction.
- As activity patterns evolve—such as training for an event—cycles can be planned for lighter weeks.

Safety and Professional Guidance

While many healthy adults tolerate periodic FMD cycles, regular monitoring ensures it remains safe and beneficial. Basic checks may include weight stability, nutrient status, and any shifts in blood pressure or glucose.

For those with underlying conditions or on medication, advance planning with a healthcare provider is essential. Even healthy individuals can benefit from periodic review to adjust calorie levels, macronutrient targets, and recovery strategies.

FMD works best when it is not an isolated, rigid event but part of a flexible, year-round approach that adapts to life's shifting demands. When applied with planning, self-awareness, and appropriate breaks, it can offer a structured window into fasting biology while leaving room for sustainable, nourishing eating the rest of the time.

FMD for Different Age Groups

The Fast Mimicking Diet (FMD) was originally developed through research in adult populations, and most clinical studies have focused on healthy middle-aged individuals. However, interest in the diet has expanded beyond this group—including younger adults, older adults, and those navigating age-specific health concerns. While the core structure of FMD remains the same, age-related differences in physiology, nutritional needs, and safety considerations require a more cautious, personalized approach.

FMD is not universally appropriate for every age group, and decisions about starting or modifying it should always be guided by a licensed healthcare provider, especially for minors, older adults, or individuals with medical conditions.

Young Adults (Ages 18–30)

Early adulthood is a period of ongoing physiological development, even after the visible milestones of adolescence have passed. Bone mass continues to build into the late twenties, and brain development — especially in regions linked to decision-making, emotional regulation, and impulse control — often extends into the mid-twenties. Many young adults also experience hormonal stabilization, which supports reproductive health, metabolic balance, and muscle development.

Activity levels in this age group can be high, whether from structured exercise, physically demanding jobs, or an active social lifestyle. For some, energy requirements are further elevated by higher lean muscle mass, long work hours, or irregular schedules such as night shifts. Nutritional needs in this stage are influenced not only by immediate energy demands but also by the long-term importance of maintaining peak bone density, preserving metabolic flexibility, and supporting reproductive and cognitive health.

Using FMD in This Life Stage

A short, occasional cycle of the Fast Mimicking Diet may be well tolerated in healthy young adults. However, it should not be approached as a routine or frequent habit without professional oversight. The potential for nutrient gaps is greater in those who repeat calorie-restricted cycles too often or without adequate recovery periods between them.

Young adults with a personal or family history of disordered eating, body image concerns, or metabolic instability (such as reactive hypoglycemia or hormonal imbalances) should be especially cautious. In these cases, structured fasting protocols, even when food is included, can sometimes reinforce restrictive patterns or create unhealthy associations with eating.

Potential Considerations

- *Higher energy demands*: Physical activity, manual labor, or irregular work hours can raise caloric and nutrient needs. Extended calorie restriction may impair performance, recovery, and general energy levels.
- *Hormonal sensitivity*: Significant calorie or protein reduction can influence menstrual regularity, fertility markers, and endocrine function in both men and women. Disruption may be more pronounced in those with existing hormonal concerns or high training volumes.
- *Psychological risks*: Using FMD primarily for appearance-driven goals increases the likelihood of unhealthy restriction patterns, especially in individuals with body image concerns or perfectionistic tendencies.
- *Nutrient priorities*: Adequate protein, calcium, vitamin D, and micronutrients are critical in this age group for supporting bone and muscle mass, immune health, and ongoing cognitive development.

A Balanced Approach

For young adults interested in supporting metabolic health, occasional FMD cycles can be combined with longer periods of balanced, plant-forward eating that meets full nutrient and calorie needs. Between cycles, meals should emphasize a variety of whole foods — vegetables, fruits, legumes, nuts, seeds, and high-quality protein sources — alongside healthy fats and adequate hydration.

Spacing FMD cycles several months apart can help protect against nutrient depletion and maintain stable energy availability for training, work, and daily activities. Aligning fasting periods with lighter activity phases or reduced physical demands may also improve tolerance and reduce the risk of performance decline.

Ultimately, in this life stage, the priority is to support growth, repair, and resilience — not to overuse fasting as a shortcut. When applied thoughtfully and infrequently, FMD may complement a well-rounded diet and lifestyle. When overused, it can interfere with the very systems that young adults need to strengthen for long-term health.

Adults in Midlife (Ages 30–55)

This age range is where FMD has the most research traction. Many individuals in their 30s, 40s, and 50s begin to see shifts in metabolism, insulin sensitivity, body composition, and inflammatory markers. These are also the decades when interest in proactive longevity strategies often begins.

In clinical studies, individuals in this demographic have shown favorable responses to multiple FMD cycles in terms of abdominal fat, fasting glucose, and some cardiovascular markers. However, the degree of benefit varies depending on baseline health status, lifestyle, and consistency.

Potential Considerations

- *Busy lifestyles* may require thoughtful planning for FMD implementation, including meal prep and recovery periods.
- *Perimenopause and menopause* in women may affect energy levels, sleep, and appetite cues during fasting cycles.
- *Medication use* (such as for blood pressure or cholesterol) may need to be adjusted, depending on how the body responds to short-term restriction.

Adults in midlife often tolerate 2–3 FMD cycles per year well, but it's important to check in with a clinician before increasing frequency or combining with other restrictive regimens like keto, intermittent fasting, or aggressive exercise.

Older Adults (Ages 60+)

With age, nutritional priorities shift to preserving muscle mass, supporting immune resilience, and avoiding frailty. These concerns may make standard FMD protocols more challenging or risky for older individuals—particularly if calorie or protein intake becomes insufficient.

While some researchers have investigated the effects of fasting and protein restriction on longevity signaling pathways in older populations, these studies are still early-stage. At this time, no standard FMD guidelines exist for individuals over 60, and the safety profile is less well established.

Potential Considerations

- *Sarcopenia* (loss of muscle mass) becomes more common with age, and insufficient protein or calorie intake—even for a few days—may contribute to further decline.
- *Hydration needs* are often higher in older adults, and fasting states can increase risk of dizziness, electrolyte imbalance, or constipation.
- *Medication interactions* are more likely, especially among those taking glucose-lowering drugs, anticoagulants, or diuretics.

For these reasons, FMD may not be recommended for older adults unless carefully supervised. If used, adjustments in calorie content, duration, or macronutrient balance may be needed to avoid adverse effects. A physician or registered dietitian should assess individual risk before attempting even a single cycle.

Teens and Adolescents (Under Age 18)

FMD is not recommended for individuals under 18. Adolescence is a critical developmental period marked by increased nutritional demands for growth, brain maturation, hormone development, and bone strength. Any form of caloric restriction during this time can disrupt these processes and pose risks to physical and psychological health.

Even teens with a high interest in nutrition or longevity science should avoid experimenting with fasting-mimicking protocols without clinical guidance. Alternative strategies that emphasize nutrient-dense meals, balanced blood sugar, and consistent eating patterns are more appropriate and sustainable for this age group.

Parents or guardians who are using FMD themselves should be mindful of how they talk about fasting, food, and weight in the household, as teens are highly sensitive to modeling behavior.

Individuals with Chronic Health Conditions

Regardless of age, individuals with chronic conditions such as diabetes, autoimmune disorders, cardiovascular disease, or gastrointestinal issues must proceed with caution. FMD is not intended to manage or treat these conditions and may affect the absorption of medications, stability of blood sugar, or symptom expression.

Certain populations may be at increased risk, including those who:

- Take insulin or sulfonylureas
- Have a history of arrhythmia or hypotension
- Experience electrolyte imbalances
- Manage GI disorders such as IBD or gastritis
- Are undergoing cancer treatment or recovering from surgery

FMD may exacerbate underlying symptoms or complicate medication protocols. In some cases, a modified, higher-calorie or shorter-duration version may be appropriate under supervision, but this should never be self-directed.

A Personalized, Age-Informed Approach

Ultimately, FMD is not a one-size-fits-all dietary intervention. What works well for a healthy 42-year-old office worker may not be suitable for a 70-year-old retiree or a 19-year-old student. Life stage, physiological demands, and clinical context all shape whether FMD is a safe or beneficial choice.

Before starting FMD at any age, it's important to ask:

- Have I ruled out any contraindications with my doctor?
- Do I have a clear reason for wanting to try this approach?
- Am I physically and mentally well enough to handle short-term restriction?

- Will I be able to eat in a nourishing, balanced way after the cycle ends?

Answering these questions honestly—and with professional input—can help ensure that FMD is approached responsibly and with full awareness of individual needs.

Foods to Eat and Avoid on the Fast Mimicking Diet

The Fast Mimicking Diet (FMD) uses a deliberate combination of lower calories, reduced protein, and specific macronutrient ratios to create many of the same physiological responses as water-only fasting—while still allowing some food intake.

These guidelines are intended as a general example of how to structure an FMD-friendly food plan. They are not therapeutic protocols and should not replace personalized recommendations from a qualified healthcare professional.

Macronutrient Targets

Research-based FMD structures generally aim for:

- *Calories*: ~700–1,100 per day (varies by body size, activity, and protocol length)
- *Carbohydrates*: 40–50% of total calories
- *Protein*: 10–15% of total calories (kept deliberately low)

- *Fats*: 40–45% of total calories (predominantly from plant-based, unsaturated sources)

These proportions help maintain enough nutrient intake to sustain daily functioning while potentially encouraging mild ketosis and temporary changes in IGF-1 levels, and other fasting-like metabolic responses.

Foods to Include

1. **Plant-Based Fats**

    High-quality plant fats make up a large share of FMD calories, providing satiety and helping the body shift into fat utilization for energy.

    - *Extra virgin olive oil* – primary fat source, rich in monounsaturated fats and polyphenols
    - *Avocado and avocado oil* – for salads, dressings, or simple toppings
    - *Nuts and seeds* – almonds, walnuts, macadamias, pecans, chia seeds, flaxseeds, pumpkin seeds
    - *Nut and seed butters* – unsweetened and minimally processed varieties
    - *Olives* – whole or sliced, as a savory addition to vegetable dishes

    Tip: Limit portions to match calorie targets—nuts and oils are calorie-dense.

2. **Low-Protein Vegetables**

Vegetables are central to FMD for fiber, micronutrients, and phytonutrients—without excessive protein that could blunt fasting signals.

- *Leafy greens* – kale, spinach, romaine, Swiss chard
- *Cruciferous vegetables* – broccoli, cauliflower, Brussels sprouts, cabbage
- *Other non-starchy vegetables* – zucchini, cucumber, peppers, celery, mushrooms
- *Sea vegetables* – nori, wakame, dulse (for iodine and minerals)

Tip: Steaming, roasting, or lightly sautéing in olive oil helps preserve nutrients while keeping digestion comfortable during low-calorie days.

3. **Moderate-Carbohydrate Vegetables & Legumes**

Small portions of starchy vegetables and legumes can provide sustained energy and help prevent excessive fatigue.

- *Root vegetables* – carrots, beets, turnips, rutabaga (avoid large servings of high-starch potatoes)
- *Winter squash* – butternut, acorn, kabocha

- ***Legumes*** – lentils, chickpeas, black beans (in limited portions to manage total protein)
- ***Green peas*** – modestly portioned to balance protein content

4. **Low-Sugar Fruits**

Fruit on FMD is used sparingly to avoid spiking glucose while still providing antioxidants and palatability.

- ***Berries*** – blueberries, raspberries, blackberries, strawberries
- ***Citrus*** – grapefruit, lemon, lime, orange segments in moderation
- ***Melons*** – cantaloupe, honeydew, watermelon (small portions)
- ***Stone fruit*** – plums, peaches, apricots (seasonal, limited amounts)

5. **Broths & Light Soups**

Broths and light vegetable soups help with hydration, electrolyte replenishment, and satiety.

- ***Vegetable broth*** – homemade or low-sodium store-bought
- ***Miso broth*** – in small amounts, as it contains sodium and trace protein
- ***Clear mushroom broth*** – rich in umami without excess calories

Avoid heavy cream-based or protein-rich soups during FMD cycles.

Foods to Limit or Avoid

The main goal is to maintain low protein and moderate carbohydrate intake while keeping calories within the set range. Foods that fall outside these parameters are best avoided during the fasting-mimicking period.

1. **High-Protein Foods**

   These can counteract fasting signals by raising IGF-1 and promoting anabolic activity.

   - Meat, poultry, fish, and seafood
   - Eggs and egg whites
   - Dairy products (milk, yogurt, cheese)
   - Protein powders, shakes, or bars

2. **Refined and High-Sugar Foods**

   These can spike blood sugar and insulin, reducing the intended fasting-like state.

   - Candy, pastries, cookies, and desserts
   - White bread, refined pasta, and most crackers
   - Sugary beverages, sodas, and sweetened teas
   - Large servings of tropical fruits (e.g., mango, pineapple, banana)

3. **Highly Processed Fats**

   Low-quality fats provide calories without beneficial nutrients.

   - Hydrogenated or partially hydrogenated oils
   - Industrial seed oils high in omega-6 (corn oil, soybean oil, cottonseed oil) when possible
   - Deep-fried foods

Hydration & Beverages

Hydration supports digestion, energy, and metabolic function during low-calorie days. Mild ketosis and reduced glycogen stores can increase fluid and electrolyte needs.

- *Water* – aim for steady intake throughout the day
- *Herbal teas* – chamomile, peppermint, ginger, rooibos, hibiscus (caffeine-free is preferable for sensitive individuals)
- *Green or black tea* – if tolerated, in moderation for a gentle caffeine lift
- *Coffee* – small amounts, ideally black or with a splash of plant-based milk; avoid high-calorie creamers and sweeteners

If lightheadedness or muscle cramping occurs, a pinch of sea salt in water or a mineral-rich broth may help—but check with your healthcare provider, especially if you have blood pressure concerns.

Supplement Considerations

FMD cycles are short, but micronutrient intake may be lower than usual. Some individuals choose to take supplements during the fasting period, while others resume them afterward. Always confirm with a healthcare professional before introducing new supplements during FMD.

Common considerations include:

- *Electrolytes* – sodium, potassium, magnesium (especially if prone to cramps or dizziness)
- *Multivitamin* – may help cover temporary gaps in micronutrient intake
- *Omega-3 fatty acids* – if not consuming fatty fish outside of FMD
- *Vitamin D* – for those with low sun exposure or deficiency risk

Structuring a Day's Intake

An example (non-prescriptive) FMD-style day might look like:

- *Morning*: Herbal tea, small portion of berries with a tablespoon of chia seeds soaked in unsweetened almond milk
- *Midday*: Steamed broccoli and zucchini drizzled with olive oil, small serving of lentils, half an avocado
- *Snack*: A few walnuts and cucumber slices

- *Evening*: Vegetable broth-based soup with kale, carrots, and mushrooms; side of roasted butternut squash with olive oil

This structure maintains the macro balance while spreading calories to avoid extreme hunger spikes.

After the FMD Cycle

Reintroduction is as important as the fasting-mimicking phase. Abruptly returning to heavy meals can cause digestive discomfort, spikes in blood sugar, and fatigue.

- Start with light, plant-based meals for the first 24 hours post-cycle
- Gradually reintroduce lean protein and higher-fiber grains
- Continue hydration and gentle movement to support digestion

The Fast Mimicking Diet works best when built around nutrient-dense, plant-forward foods that match its specific macronutrient goals. Choosing whole ingredients, staying well hydrated, and pacing reintroduction after the cycle can help support comfort and adherence. With mindful planning and professional guidance, these guidelines can be adapted to individual preferences and needs.

The Two-Week Fast Mimicking Diet Plan

The Fast Mimicking Diet (FMD) works best when approached as a *short, purposeful cycle* rather than a sudden, high-restriction shock to the body. Easing into the process helps you adapt physically and mentally, reducing discomfort and improving follow-through.

This two-week structure allows for a *gradual entry* in Week 1, a *targeted fasting-mimicking phase* in Week 2, and a careful transition back to normal eating. While some research uses a 5-day FMD window, adding a preparation week can make the experience more sustainable and less stressful.

Week 1 – Preparation & Adaptation

Week 1 is your launchpad. You're not fasting yet — you're getting your body, kitchen, and schedule ready. This is when you fine-tune eating patterns, reduce certain triggers, and begin shifting toward the macronutrient ratios you'll follow more strictly in Week 2.

1. **Calorie Tapering**

   Rather than cutting from your usual intake directly to 700–1,100 kcal, reduce gradually.

   A *10–20% calorie reduction* is a comfortable target for most adults.

   - If you normally eat ~2,000 kcal, drop to ~1,600–1,800 kcal.
   - This gentler start trains your appetite to accept smaller portions.

   During this stage, pay attention to:

   - *Hunger patterns* — notice if you tend to eat out of habit, boredom, or emotion.
   - *Satiety foods* — see which meals keep you fuller with fewer calories.
   - *Mood shifts* — some people feel irritable when cutting back too abruptly; tapering helps.

2. **Macronutrient Adjustment**

   Start moving toward the FMD balance:

   - *Carbohydrates*: 45–50%
   - *Protein*: 15–20%
   - *Fat*: 30–35%

   Protein remains slightly higher than in Week 2 to maintain satiety and muscle support while adapting.

Example Day (~1,750 kcal):

- *Breakfast*: Steel-cut oats cooked in almond milk, topped with blueberries, chia seeds, and a drizzle of almond butter.
- *Lunch*: Quinoa, chickpea, cucumber, tomato, parsley, olive oil, and lemon salad.
- *Snack*: Apple slices with a few raw almonds.
- *Dinner*: Roasted sweet potato, steamed broccoli, and a small portion of grilled tofu.

3. **Caffeine & Sugar Taper**

One hidden challenge of FMD isn't the calorie restriction itself — it's withdrawal from caffeine or sugar if you rely on them daily. Sudden removal can cause headaches, fatigue, or irritability.

- If you drink three cups of coffee, taper to one or two by the end of Week 1.
- Begin swapping refined sweets for fruit or naturally sweet root vegetables.

4. **Hydration Habits**

Increase fluid intake to *at least 2 liters daily*. Mild dehydration can amplify fatigue during FMD. Herbal teas — peppermint, chamomile, rooibos — provide variety without adding calories or stimulants.

5. **Environment & Meal Prep**

   Clear your pantry of highly processed snacks that might tempt you during Week 2. Shop for fresh produce, healthy fats (avocado, nuts, olive oil), and low-protein plant foods you'll use in FMD meals. Prepping ahead removes decision fatigue and keeps you on track.

Week 2 – Core FMD Phase

This is the main fasting-mimicking window — *five consecutive days* of low-calorie, low-protein, high-fat, plant-forward eating, framed within a week that also includes light entry and recovery days.

<u>**Targets for Core Days (Days 2–6 of Week 2):**</u>

- Calories: ~700–1,100 kcal
- Carbohydrates: 40–50%
- Protein: 10–15%
- Fat: 40–45%

These ranges are designed to send metabolic signals similar to fasting while still providing some fuel for daily functioning.

1. **Meal Timing**

   Most people do well on *two or three small meals* spaced through the day.

- A 10–12 hour eating window (e.g., 8 a.m. to 6 p.m.) can align with circadian rhythms without layering on the extra challenge of full intermittent fasting.
- Avoid constant grazing — the body benefits from clear breaks between meals.

2. Food Selection

The goal is low-protein, plant-based foods rich in fiber and healthy fats, with moderate complex carbs.

Foundations:

- *Vegetables*: Non-starchy and starchy — zucchini, spinach, cauliflower, carrots, beets, sweet potato.
- *Healthy fats*: Olive oil, avocado, nuts, seeds, tahini.
- *Complex carbs*: Quinoa, buckwheat, lentils (in small amounts to keep protein low).
- *Flavors*: Herbs, spices, lemon, and vinegar for interest without adding protein.

3. Example FMD Day (~900 kcal)

Breakfast: Steamed spinach and zucchini drizzled with olive oil; a small roasted sweet potato. (~250 kcal)

Lunch: Vegetable soup (carrots, celery, cabbage) with olive oil; avocado slices on the side. (~350 kcal)

Snack: A small handful of walnuts. (~150 kcal)

Dinner: Roasted beets, cauliflower, and carrots with tahini-lemon sauce. (~200 kcal)

4. **Activity Level**

Keep physical activity gentle:

- Walking, stretching, or restorative yoga.
- Avoid intense workouts; low glycogen stores can make strenuous exercise feel harder and may increase fatigue risk.

5. **Managing Hunger**

Day 1–2 can feel challenging as the body transitions. By Day 3, many people notice hunger subsides and mental clarity increases.

- Hydration is key — drink water or herbal tea between meals.
- Mindful eating helps maximize satisfaction from smaller portions.

Recovery & Transition (Days 7–8 of Week 2)

After the low-calorie days, it's tempting to celebrate with a large meal — but this can cause digestive upset. A *gentle reintroduction* of calories and protein is more comfortable.

Day 7

- Add 200–300 kcal over FMD levels, focusing on vegetables, fruit, and small portions of lean plant proteins like lentils or tofu.
- Continue healthy fats for energy stability.

Day 8

- Increase toward normal calorie intake.
- Gradually reintroduce your usual protein level.
- Bring back whole grains, legumes, and (if part of your diet) animal proteins in moderate amounts.

Key Considerations for Both Weeks

1. *Medical Guidance*: Anyone with chronic conditions, on medication, pregnant, breastfeeding, underweight, or with a history of eating disorders should only attempt FMD under professional supervision.
2. *Listening to Your Body*: Mild hunger or reduced energy is expected, but dizziness, extreme fatigue, or other concerning symptoms are a signal to stop and seek medical advice.
3. *Tracking Your Experience*: Journaling energy, mood, sleep quality, and digestion can help you decide if and how to repeat FMD. Physical measures like waist circumference or body composition can be added if relevant.

4. ***Frequency***: Clinical research often uses FMD 2–3 times per year, but the ideal frequency varies. Always adjust based on personal tolerance and professional input.

Why the Two-Week Structure Works

The preparation week smooths the entry into calorie restriction, reducing the "shock" factor of starting at 700–1,100 kcal. It also helps identify any logistical or emotional barriers before you're deep into the process. The recovery phase ensures you transition safely, avoiding digestive distress and stabilizing your energy as you return to regular eating.

By treating FMD as a *cycle* — prepare, mimic, recover — the experience feels more deliberate and less like a crash diet, which supports both comfort and long-term adherence.

Sample Recipes

Below are a plant-forward, low-protein recipe section you can adapt for the FMD guide. Each is built with whole ingredients, healthy fats, and moderate complex carbohydrates—avoiding any proprietary or branded formulas—while keeping protein modest.

Kale Lentil Bowl

A warm, earthy meal that's both filling and light.

Serves: 1 | **Calories**: ~280 kcal | **Carbs**: 38g | **Protein**: 8g | **Fat**: 12g

FMD Core Day Adjustment: Lentils are higher in protein, so reduce to 2–3 tablespoons cooked during the fasting-mimicking phase to help maintain the low-protein target.

Ingredients:

- 1 cup chopped kale
- ½ cup cooked green lentils (see adjustment note above)
- ½ cup roasted sweet potato cubes
- 1 tsp olive oil
- ½ tsp lemon juice
- Pinch of smoked paprika

Instructions:

1. Lightly steam kale until tender, about 3–4 minutes.
2. In a medium bowl, combine kale, lentils, and sweet potato.

3. Drizzle with olive oil and lemon juice, then sprinkle with smoked paprika.
4. Toss gently and serve warm.

This bowl is rich in fiber and slow-digesting carbs, with just enough healthy fat to keep energy steady during FMD days.

Zucchini & Olive Salad

A crisp, hydrating dish with a savory kick.

Serves: 1 | **Calories**: ~220 kcal | **Carbs**: 14g | **Protein**: 4g | **Fat**: 18g

Ingredients:

- 1 medium zucchini, spiralized or thinly sliced
- 6 kalamata olives, sliced
- ½ cup cherry tomatoes, halved
- 1 tsp extra virgin olive oil
- 1 tsp apple cider vinegar
- Pinch of dried oregano

Instructions:

1. Combine zucchini, olives, and tomatoes in a salad bowl.
2. Whisk olive oil, vinegar, and oregano until blended.
3. Pour dressing over vegetables, toss gently, and chill for 10 minutes before eating.

Perfect for a light lunch or side, this salad offers hydrating vegetables, heart-healthy fats, and a pop of acidity to awaken the palate.

Roasted Cauliflower with Tahini Drizzle

Nutty, creamy, and satisfying without being heavy.

Serves: 1 | **Calories**: ~260 kcal | **Carbs**: 18g | **Protein**: 6g | **Fat**: 20g

Ingredients:

- 1½ cups cauliflower florets
- 1 tsp olive oil
- 1 tbsp tahini
- 1 tsp lemon juice
- Pinch of cumin

Instructions:

1. Preheat the oven to 400°F (200°C). Toss cauliflower with olive oil and roast for 20–25 minutes until golden.
2. In a small bowl, whisk tahini, lemon juice, cumin, and 1–2 tsp water until smooth.
3. Arrange roasted cauliflower on a plate, drizzle with sauce, and serve warm.

This dish offers satisfying texture and flavor while keeping protein low, making it ideal for FMD core days.

Sweet Potato & Walnut Mash

Comforting and slightly sweet with a nutty crunch.

Serves: 1 | *Calories*: ~300 kcal | *Carbs*: 36g | *Protein*: 4g | *Fat*: 18g

Ingredients:

- 1 small sweet potato, peeled and cubed
- 2 tsp olive oil
- 1 tbsp finely chopped walnuts
- Pinch of cinnamon

Instructions:

1. Steam sweet potato until tender, about 10–12 minutes.
2. Mash with olive oil until smooth.
3. Sprinkle it with walnuts and cinnamon before serving.

This simple recipe provides slow-release carbs for gentle energy and brain-boosting omega-3s from the walnuts.

Spinach Avocado Wrap

A portable, nutrient-packed meal with creamy texture.

Serves: 1 | **Calories**: ~270 kcal | **Carbs**: 28g | **Protein**: 5g | **Fat**: 16g

Ingredients:

- 1 small whole-grain tortilla (~6")
- ½ small avocado, sliced
- 1 cup baby spinach
- 2 slices roasted red pepper
- ½ tsp lemon juice

Instructions:

1. Lay the tortilla flat and arrange spinach, avocado, and red pepper in the center.
2. Drizzle with lemon juice for freshness.
3. Roll tightly, slice in half, and serve immediately.

A great on-the-go option that's balanced in carbs and fats, supporting steady energy during low-calorie days.

Cucumber & Avocado Salad

Cool, creamy, and refreshing for light meals.

Serves: 1 | **Calories**: ~210 kcal | **Carbs**: 12g | **Protein**: 3g | **Fat**: 17g

Ingredients:

- 1 cup diced cucumber
- ½ small avocado, cubed
- 1 tbsp chopped parsley
- 1 tsp olive oil
- ½ tsp lemon juice
- Pinch of sea salt

Instructions:

1. Combine cucumber, avocado, and parsley in a bowl.
2. Whisk olive oil and lemon juice; drizzle over salad.
3. Toss gently, season with salt, and serve immediately.

This salad is high in hydration and healthy fats, making it satisfying without overloading on calories.

Roasted Carrots with Sesame

Sweet with a nutty finish.

Serves: 1 | **Calories**: ~240 kcal | **Carbs**: 26g | **Protein**: 4g | **Fat**: 14g

Ingredients:

- 1 cup carrot sticks
- 1 tsp olive oil
- 1 tsp sesame seeds
- Pinch of ground coriander

Instructions:

1. Preheat the oven to 375°F (190°C). Toss carrots with olive oil and coriander.
2. Roast for 20–25 minutes until tender.
3. Sprinkle with sesame seeds before serving.

An easy side dish that delivers carotenoids for eye health while keeping protein minimal.

Warm Quinoa & Vegetable Bowl

(Contains quinoa — limit portion on core FMD days)

Hearty yet light, perfect for lunch or dinner.

Serves: 1 | **Calories**: ~300 kcal | **Carbs**: 40g | **Protein**: 6g | **Fat**: 12g

Ingredients:

- ½ cup cooked quinoa (reduce to 2–3 tbsp cooked on core FMD days to maintain low protein target)
- ½ cup steamed broccoli
- ¼ cup roasted red peppers
- 1 tsp olive oil
- Pinch of black pepper

Instructions:

1. In a medium bowl, combine quinoa, broccoli, and red peppers.
2. Drizzle with olive oil, season with pepper, and toss gently.
3. Serve warm, or let cool slightly for a room-temperature meal.

Provides balanced complex carbs, antioxidants from vegetables, and healthy fats to sustain energy.

Eggplant with Garlic Tahini Sauce

Silky, rich, and full of flavor.

Serves: 1 | **Calories**: ~280 kcal | **Carbs**: 18g | **Protein**: 5g | **Fat**: 20g

Ingredients:

- 1 cup diced eggplant
- 1 tsp olive oil
- 1 tbsp tahini
- ½ small garlic clove, minced
- 1 tsp lemon juice

Instructions:

1. Roast eggplant at 400°F (200°C) for 20 minutes until tender.
2. Mix tahini, garlic, lemon juice, and 1–2 tsp water until smooth.
3. Plate eggplant and drizzle sauce over the top.

A nutrient-dense dish with creamy texture and a savory garlic kick.

Tomato & Basil Zoodle Bowl

A light, pasta-like meal without the heaviness.

Serves: 1 | **Calories**: ~190 kcal | **Carbs**: 20g | **Protein**: 4g | **Fat**: 10g

Ingredients:

- 1 medium zucchini, spiralized
- ½ cup cherry tomatoes, halved
- 1 tsp olive oil
- 3–4 basil leaves, torn
- Pinch of black pepper

Instructions:

1. Sauté zucchini noodles in olive oil for 1–2 minutes until just tender.
2. Toss with tomatoes and basil.
3. Season with pepper and serve immediately.

A fresh, quick option that's high in water content and easy on digestion.

Steamed Broccoli with Almond Drizzle

Simple, satisfying, and full of micronutrients.

Serves: 1 | **Calories**: ~200 kcal | **Carbs**: 12g | **Protein**: 5g | **Fat**: 15g

Ingredients:

- 1 cup broccoli florets
- 1 tsp almond butter
- 1 tsp olive oil
- 1 tsp lemon juice

Instructions:

1. Steam broccoli until tender-crisp, about 5 minutes.
2. Whisk almond butter, olive oil, and lemon juice until smooth.
3. Drizzle over broccoli before serving.

Combines healthy fats and fiber for lasting fullness.

Beet & Orange Salad

Bright, slightly sweet, and refreshing.

Serves: 1 | **Calories**: ~230 kcal | **Carbs**: 26g | **Protein**: 4g | **Fat**: 14g

Ingredients:
- 1 cup cooked, diced beets
- ½ small orange, segmented
- 1 tsp olive oil
- 1 tsp balsamic vinegar
- Pinch of ground cinnamon

Instructions:
1. In a bowl, combine beets and orange segments.
2. Whisk olive oil, vinegar, and cinnamon; pour over salad.
3. Toss gently and serve chilled.

A colorful dish packed with antioxidants and natural sweetness.

Roasted Brussels Sprouts with Lemon Oil

Crisp-edged and bright with citrus.

Serves: 1 | **Calories**: ~210 kcal | **Carbs**: 18g | **Protein**: 5g | **Fat**: 14g

Ingredients:

- 1 cup halved Brussels sprouts
- 1 tsp olive oil
- 1 tsp lemon juice
- Pinch of sea salt and black pepper

Instructions:

1. Preheat the oven to 400°F (200°C). Toss sprouts with olive oil, salt, and pepper.
2. Roast for 20–25 minutes, shaking the pan halfway.
3. Drizzle with lemon juice before serving.

A high-fiber side that's easy to prepare and adds variety to FMD vegetable rotation.

Mediterranean Chickpea Salad

Light, fresh, and satisfying.

FMD note: Chickpeas are higher in protein, so use a smaller portion (about 2–3 tablespoons cooked) on core FMD days to stay within low-protein targets.

Serves: 1 | **Calories**: ~250 kcal | **Carbs**: 28g | **Protein**: 7g | **Fat**: 12g

Ingredients:

- ½ cup cooked chickpeas (reduce to 2–3 tbsp on core FMD days)
- ½ cup cucumber, diced
- ½ cup cherry tomatoes, halved
- 1 tsp olive oil
- ½ tsp red wine vinegar
- Pinch of oregano

Instructions:

1. Combine chickpeas, cucumber, and tomatoes in a bowl.
2. Whisk olive oil, vinegar, and oregano; pour over salad.
3. Toss gently and chill before serving.

Provides steady energy with a balance of fiber, healthy fats, and modest protein.

Roasted Red Pepper & Almond Dip

Smooth and flavorful, great with vegetable sticks.

Serves: 1 | **Calories**: ~230 kcal | **Carbs**: 12g | **Protein**: 4g | **Fat**: 18g

Ingredients:

- ½ cup roasted red peppers (jarred, rinsed)
- 1 tbsp almonds
- 1 tsp olive oil
- ½ tsp lemon juice

Instructions:

1. Blend all ingredients until smooth.
2. Adjust seasoning with salt if desired.
3. Serve with cucumber sticks, celery, or zucchini rounds.

A versatile dip that fits well into snack times on FMD days.

Spiced Pumpkin Soup

Warm, smooth, and naturally sweet.

Serves: 1 | **Calories**: ~240 kcal | **Carbs**: 32g | **Protein**: 4g | **Fat**: 12g

Ingredients:

- 1 cup pumpkin puree
- 1 cup vegetable broth (low sodium)
- 1 tsp olive oil
- ¼ tsp ground ginger
- Pinch of cinnamon

Instructions:

1. Heat olive oil in a pot, stir in pumpkin puree.
2. Add broth, ginger, and cinnamon; simmer for 5 minutes.
3. Blend for extra smoothness if desired.

A comforting bowl with slow-release carbs and gentle spices that support digestion.

These recipes offer variety, balanced flavors, and nutrient-dense ingredients to support both the preparation and core phases of the Fast Mimicking Diet. By focusing on vegetables, healthy fats, and modest complex carbohydrates, they align with the diet's macronutrient goals while keeping meals enjoyable. With simple preparation and flexible pairings, they can fit easily into a sustainable FMD routine.

Conclusion

The Fast Mimicking Diet (FMD) represents a structured approach designed to help individuals experience some of the metabolic changes observed with fasting—without requiring complete food deprivation. By carefully modulating calorie intake and adjusting macronutrient ratios over a short period, FMD provides an alternative to traditional fasting that may be more accessible and sustainable for some people, supporting temporary shifts in metabolic processes.

Throughout this guide, we've explored the science behind FMD, the mechanisms it taps into (such as ketosis, autophagy, and IGF-1 reduction), and how it differs from other fasting strategies like intermittent fasting. It is important to remember that while FMD may offer promising benefits, such as potential support for healthy aging, metabolic flexibility, and cellular stress resilience, individual responses can vary. What works for one person may not have the same effect on another, and it's essential to approach this or any dietary intervention with realistic expectations.

As with any dietary or lifestyle change, FMD is not a one-size-fits-all solution. We've highlighted key considerations, such as the importance of individualized medical guidance, especially for those with underlying health conditions or specific dietary needs. The success of FMD relies not just on following the meal plan but also on understanding how it fits into your personal health journey. For some, it may complement broader health goals; for others, it may not be the best fit.

This guide has also offered practical tools for implementing FMD, from meal plans and recipes to tips for managing the psychological and emotional challenges that can arise during periods of caloric restriction. The insights on cravings, emotional regulation, and mindful eating serve as helpful strategies to ensure the experience is not just physically sustainable, but emotionally manageable as well.

FMD is not intended as a long-term eating pattern but as a short-term dietary approach that may be repeated periodically, ideally under medical or qualified health professional supervision—especially for individuals with existing health conditions or on medication. Whether the goal is weight management, supporting aspects of metabolic function, or exploring the potential effects of fasting-mimicking strategies, FMD provides a structured framework that can be adapted to different personal needs and preferences.

Thank you for taking the time to read this guide. By now, you have a clearer understanding of how the Fast Mimicking Diet works, how it might benefit you, and how to approach it in a safe and informed manner. If you choose to embark on this dietary journey, we encourage you to listen to your body, track your experiences, and consult a healthcare provider to ensure that this approach supports your long-term well-being.

We hope this guide has provided you with the tools, knowledge, and confidence to make an informed decision about whether FMD aligns with your health goals. Keep in mind that your health journey is unique—FMD is just one potential tool to help you navigate it. Best of luck as you explore how this structured approach may support your metabolic health and overall wellness.

Frequently Asked Questions

Is it safe for people with diabetes, high blood pressure, or postmenopausal women?

Research on the Fast Mimicking Diet (FMD) has involved a variety of adults, but safety depends heavily on personal health circumstances, current medications, and nutritional needs.

For those managing diabetes, changes in calorie and carbohydrate intake can affect blood sugar, sometimes requiring medication adjustments. People with high blood pressure may experience shifts in fluid balance or blood pressure control during calorie restriction. Postmenopausal women may have additional considerations around bone health, hormonal balance, and metabolism. In all these situations, the decision to try FMD should be made in partnership with a healthcare provider who can tailor the plan to individual needs.

Can I exercise during FMD?

Many people find they can maintain light or moderate activity such as walking, stretching, or yoga while following FMD, though the reduced calorie intake can make high-intensity exercise more taxing.

It's worth paying attention to energy levels, resting more when needed, and ensuring hydration remains consistent. If your normal routine includes vigorous training, it may be more comfortable to scale back during the diet and resume intense sessions afterward. Your doctor can help you decide what is safe based on your current health and fitness.

What if I get hungry?

Feeling some hunger—especially in the first couple of days—is common. Staying hydrated with water or unsweetened herbal tea can help, as can spacing small meals throughout the day rather than eating all calories in one sitting.

Some people find that light activity, reading, or engaging in a hobby distracts from temporary hunger signals. If hunger is severe, brings on dizziness, or causes symptoms like rapid heartbeat or confusion, it's important to stop and seek medical advice rather than trying to push through discomfort.

How often can I do FMD per year?

There is no universal schedule for how often to repeat FMD. In studies, some people have completed cycles monthly while others do it only a few times a year, depending on their goals, health status, and how well they recover between cycles.

Nutritional status, body composition, and existing health conditions all influence how often it may be safe or beneficial. A healthcare professional can help establish an appropriate frequency and ensure you are meeting nutrient needs between cycles.

Can I drink coffee during FMD?

Black coffee or coffee with minimal additives is sometimes included in reduced-calorie eating patterns, but caffeine can influence hunger, hydration, and digestion. While some find it helps manage appetite, others may feel jittery or have disrupted sleep.

It's worth discussing coffee intake with your healthcare provider, especially if you have heart rhythm concerns, high blood pressure, or anxiety, and considering herbal teas or caffeine-free options if you notice unwanted effects.

What happens after the FMD cycle ends?

Transitioning back to regular eating is an important part of the process. Shifting too quickly to large portions or highly processed foods can lead to digestive discomfort or rapid fluid changes.

Many people find it helpful to ease back in with balanced meals that include whole grains, vegetables, lean protein sources, and healthy fats. Using the period after FMD to reinforce nutrient-rich eating habits can support overall well-being between cycles.

Can FMD be done while traveling or during busy work weeks?

The reduced calorie and specific macronutrient balance of FMD can make it challenging to follow without planning. Preparing simple, portable meals in advance, keeping hydration in mind, and avoiding social situations centered around food can help.

Still, many find it easier to schedule FMD during a week when they have more control over their environment. If travel or demanding schedules can't be avoided, a healthcare provider can help adapt the approach so it remains safe and sustainable.

References and Helpful Links

Longo & Mattson (2015) — A landmark study in Cell Metabolism introducing the FMD showed that a structured low-calorie, low-protein, moderate-carb diet lowers glucose and IGF-1 while raising ketones USC Leonard Davis School of Gerontology+15AIIO+15Biology Insights+15USC Leonard Davis School of Gerontology+8Cell+8Wikipedia+8.

Pilot Human Trial (2015) — In a small human pilot, three monthly 5-day FMD cycles produced favorable shifts in aging, diabetes, cardiovascular, and cancer biomarkers with no major side effects USC Stem Cell+4USC Leonard Davis School of Gerontology+4JAMA Network+4.

JAMA Clinical Trial — Participants who completed three consecutive monthly FMD cycles (versus controls) saw reductions in body weight (≈6 lb), trunk fat, waist circumference, blood pressure, and IGF-1 levels ScienceDaily+15JAMA Network+15The Sun+15.

Nature Communications (2024) — A USC-led study demonstrated that FMD cycles reduced insulin resistance, liver fat, immune system aging, and even biological age in humans USC Stem Cell+1.

Systematic Review & Meta-Analysis (2025) — Eleven RCTs examining FMD's impact on cardiovascular risk markers found significant reductions in HbA1c, IGF-1, systolic and diastolic blood pressure Fondazione Valter Longo+15BioMed Central+15Business Insider+15.

Cardiometabolic & Sensory Outcomes — Six monthly FMD cycles, followed by normal eating, improved taste/smell function and reduced cardiometabolic and inflammatory markers in overweight individuals JAMA Network+8Cell+8USC Stem Cell+8.

Mediterranean Diet Comparison — A randomized trial comparing four monthly FMD cycles vs. a continuous Mediterranean diet assessed effects on endothelial function and vascular compliance Nature+1.

Nutrition Reviews (2025 Narrative Review) — Summarizes periodic FMD's implications for healthspan, lifespan, and multiple chronic conditions while highlighting adherence challenges and rebound risks Oxford Academic.

Bibliometric Study (2024, Frontiers in Nutrition) — Surveys the growing scholarly interest and publishing trends related to FMD Frontiers.

Metabolic Mechanisms — FMD engages pathways involved in autophagy, reduced IGF-1 signaling, and ketone rise—the hallmarks of fasting metabolism arxiv.org+15Cell+15AACR Journals+15.

Broader Evidence — Reviews of intermittent fasting and calorie restriction offer context for FMD, noting its relative sustainability and early safety profile for healthy individuals Wikipedia+15Wikipedia+15GQ+15.

www.ingramcontent.com/pod-product-compliance
Lightning Source LLC
LaVergne TN
LVHW012028060526
838201LV00061B/4516